HEART ATTACK SURVIVORS GUIDE

ROADMAP TO RECOVERY
AND PREVENTION

Dr A MITRA MBBS, MD, DMI

Disclaimer:

The information provided in this book is intended for educational purposes only. While every effort has been made to ensure accuracy and relevance, readers are advised to consult healthcare professionals for personalized advice and treatment options tailored to individual circumstances. The author and publisher disclaim any liability arising directly or indirectly from the use or application of the contents of this book.

Copyright © 2024 Dr A Mitra

All rights reserved.

ISBN:

DEDICATION

To the Reader,

I may never meet you, but this book is dedicated to you. In the quiet moments of your life, when you seek hope and strength, may these pages be a companion to your journey. You have faced the unimaginable, and your courage is boundless. This book is a testament to your resilience, your will to thrive, and your commitment to living well after a heart attack.

Every word is written with you in mind, with the hope that it brings you comfort, knowledge, and inspiration. You are not alone. Your story of recovery, healing, and living fully is woven into every chapter. May you find in these pages a beacon of light, guiding you to a future filled with health, happiness, and endless possibilities.

With all my heart,

Dr A Mitra

HEART ATTACK SURVIVORS GUIDE

CONTENTS

Part 1: Understanding Heart Attack

1	The Healing Journey Begins	3
2	The Science Behind The Scar	9
3	Facing Treatment Options	13

Part 2: Building A Foundation For A Healthy Heart

4	Partnering With Your Doctor	17
5	Diet For Heart Health	22
6	Moving Forward After A Heart Attack	27
7	Healing Through Movement	32
8	Taming The Stress Tiger	36

Part 3: Risk Factor Reduction - A Lifelong Commitment

9	Cholesterol Control	40
10	Blood Pressure Matters	44
11	Weight Management	49
12	Smoking Cessation	54

13	Diabetes And Heart Health	58

Part 4: Living A Fulfilling Life After A Heart Attack

14	Returning To Work And Activity	62
15	Sleep And Heart Health	66
16	Building Resilience	71
17	The Power Of Support	75
18	Sex And Intimacy After A Heart Attack	79

Part 5: Looking Forward - A Lifetime Of Heart Health

19	Prevention Is Key	83
20	Staying Motivated	89
21	Celebrating Success	93
22	Living With Gratitude	97
23	Empowering Yourself With Knowledge	101

ACKNOWLEDGMENTS

Creating this book has been a journey filled with the invaluable support and expertise of many individuals. I am profoundly grateful to the patients and caregivers who shared their experiences, the medical professionals and heart attack specialists who provided crucial information, and my editorial team for their meticulous work. To my family and friends, thank you for your constant encouragement and understanding. This book is dedicated to all those living after a heart attack and their caregivers, with the hope that it offers the support and information needed to navigate this journey with hope and strength.

PART 1: UNDERSTANDING HEART ATTACK

CHAPTER 1: THE HEALING JOURNEY BEGINS

Understanding the Heart Attack: A Journey Through Your Body

Imagine your heart as a powerful pump, constantly working to send blood throughout your body. This blood carries oxygen, the fuel your cells need to function properly. But the heart itself also needs oxygen-rich blood to keep pumping strong. This vital oxygen delivery happens through tiny tubes called coronary arteries, like highways delivering oxygenated blood directly to the heart muscle.

A heart attack occurs when one of these coronary arteries gets blocked, preventing enough oxygen-rich blood from reaching a part of the heart muscle. This blockage is often caused by a buildup of fatty deposits called plaque lining the inside walls of the arteries. Over time, plaque can narrow the arteries, reducing blood flow. In some cases, a piece of plaque can rupture and form a blood clot that completely blocks the artery.

When a blockage occurs, the heart muscle beyond that point is starved of oxygen. This oxygen deprivation damages the heart muscle cells, and if blood flow is not restored quickly, the affected area can die. The dead tissue eventually forms a scar.

The Warning Signs

While not everyone experiences the same symptoms, there are some common signs that might indicate a heart attack:

- **Chest pain or pressure:** This could feel like a tightness, squeezing, or burning sensation in your chest. It is often described as an uncomfortable pressure like someone sitting on your chest.

- **Pain radiating to other areas:** The pain may spread to your arm, shoulder, back, jaw, or teeth.

- **Feeling short of breath:** You might feel a sudden difficulty breathing or shortness of breath, even when you are at rest.

- **Cold sweat:** Breaking out in a cold sweat can be a sign of a heart attack, especially if accompanied by other symptoms.

- **Nausea or vomiting:** Feeling sick to your stomach or actually vomiting can occur during a heart attack.

- **Lightheadedness or dizziness:** You might feel faint or dizzy, like you might pass out.

Seeking Immediate Medical Attention

A heart attack is a medical emergency. If you experience any of the symptoms listed above, especially chest pain, your local emergency number immediately. Do not wait to see if the symptoms go away. The sooner you get medical attention, the less damage to your heart muscle. Early intervention can significantly improve your chances of a full recovery.

The Healing Process

Once you receive medical attention, your doctor will work to restore blood flow to the affected area and minimize further damage. Depending on the severity of the blockage, treatment might involve medications to dissolve blood clots, procedures to open the blocked artery (angioplasty or bypass surgery), or a combination of both.

After the initial treatment, your body begins the healing process. The white blood cells clean up the dead tissue, and over time, your body replaces it with scar tissue. While scar tissue is strong, it is not as flexible as healthy heart muscle. This can affect the heart's pumping efficiency, but with proper lifestyle changes and medications, you can still live a long and healthy life after a heart attack.

Understanding a Heart Attack empowers you to take control of your health. You can reduce your risk of heart attack by following a heart-healthy diet, exercising regularly, maintaining a healthy weight, managing stress, and not smoking. By making these changes and working with your doctor, you can protect your heart and enjoy an active and fulfilling life.

The Emotional Rollercoaster: Navigating the Feelings After a Heart Attack

A heart attack is not just a physical event; it is an emotional rollercoaster. It can leave you feeling scared, anxious, angry, and even depressed. This is completely normal. Here is why:

Facing Your Mortality: A heart attack can be a stark reminder of your own mortality. You might wonder, "What if I hadn't made it?" This can lead to feelings of fear and anxiety about the future.

Loss of Control: You might feel a loss of control over your own body. You relied on your heart to function perfectly, and now you have experienced a setback. This can be frustrating and lead to feelings of helplessness.

Grief and Anger: You might experience a sense of grief for the life you had before the heart attack. You might have to make changes to your lifestyle, which can feel like a loss. This can lead to anger, both at yourself and the situation.

Depression: The physical limitations and changes brought on by a heart attack can be discouraging. You might feel down and lose interest in activities you once enjoyed. These are all symptoms of depression, which is a common occurrence after a heart attack.

Coping with Change: A heart attack can force you to make significant changes to your lifestyle. This can be stressful, especially if you are not used to a structured routine. Adapting to new dietary habits and exercise programs can be challenging.

Do not Go Through It Alone

It is important to remember that you are not alone in experiencing these emotions. Here are some ways to navigate this emotional rollercoaster:

Talk to Your Doctor: Your doctor cannot just treat the physical aspects of a heart attack; they can also address the emotional impact. Talk openly about your fears and anxieties. They might recommend therapy or support groups to help you cope.

Talk to Loved Ones: Do not bottle up your emotions. Talk to your family and friends about how you are feeling. Their support and understanding can make a huge difference.

Join a Support Group: Connecting with others who have experienced a heart attack can be incredibly helpful. Sharing your feelings with people who understand what you are going through can be very validating.

Focus on Self-Care: Taking care of yourself emotionally is just as important as taking care of yourself physically. Make time for relaxation techniques like deep breathing or meditation. Find healthy ways to manage stress, like spending time in nature or listening to calming music.

Celebrate Your Victories: Recovery is a journey, not a destination. Focus on the small wins, like completing a short walk or mastering a new recipe. Celebrating these achievements keeps you motivated and fosters a positive outlook.

Remember, a heart attack does not define you. By acknowledging your emotions, seeking support, and prioritizing self-care, you can navigate the emotional impact of a heart attack and move forward with a positive and hopeful attitude.

CHAPTER 2: THE SCIENCE BEHIND THE SCAR

How Heart Attacks Happen and Heal

After a heart attack, it is natural to wonder what happened inside your body. This chapter dives into the science behind your recovery, explaining how heart attacks occur and how your body heals.

The Mighty Heart and its Lifelines

Imagine your heart as a powerful fist-sized muscle that tirelessly pumps blood throughout your body. This blood carries oxygen, the fuel your cells need to function. Just like any hard worker needs energy, your heart muscle itself also needs oxygen-rich blood to keep going.

To deliver this vital oxygen, your heart has tiny highways called coronary arteries. These arteries branch off from a larger artery called the aorta and encircle your heart like a crown. Think of these arteries as delivery trucks bringing oxygen-rich blood directly to the heart muscle.

The Blockage and the Damage

A heart attack happens when one of these coronary arteries gets blocked. This blockage is often caused by a buildup of fatty deposits called plaque lining the inside walls of the arteries. Over time, this plaque can narrow the arteries, reducing the amount of blood that can flow through. In some cases, a piece of plaque might rupture and form a blood clot that completely blocks the artery.

When a blockage occurs, the heart muscle beyond that point is starved of oxygen. This oxygen deprivation causes damage to the heart muscle cells. If blood flow is not restored quickly, the affected area can die. The dead tissue eventually forms a scar.

Understanding Your Risk Factors

Several factors can increase your risk of developing plaque buildup and having a heart attack. These include:

- **High cholesterol:** High levels of LDL cholesterol, also known as "bad" cholesterol, contribute to plaque formation.

- **High blood pressure:** Uncontrolled blood pressure puts extra strain on your heart and arteries, damaging them over time.

- **Smoking:** Smoking damages the lining of your arteries and increases your risk of blood clots.

- **Diabetes:** Diabetes can damage blood vessels and increase the risk of plaque buildup.

- **Family history:** Having a family history of heart disease increases your risk.

- **Being overweight or obese:** Excess weight puts a strain on your heart and increases your risk of other conditions like diabetes and high blood pressure.

The Healing Process: From Damage to Scar Tissue

Your body starts healing the damaged area right after the heart attack. Your white blood cells rush to the site of the injury, cleaning up the dead tissue. Over time, your body replaces the dead tissue with scar tissue. This scar tissue is strong but less flexible than healthy heart muscle. While it allows the heart to continue functioning, it can affect its pumping efficiency.

Treatment Options Overview

The treatment options for a heart attack depend on the severity of the blockage and the extent of the damage. Here is a brief overview:

- **Medications:** Medications can help dissolve blood clots, lower cholesterol levels, and improve blood flow to the heart.

- **Angioplasty:** This procedure involves inserting a tiny balloon into the blocked artery to open it up. Sometimes a stent, a small wire mesh tube, is placed in the artery to keep it open.

- **Bypass surgery:** In this surgery, a healthy blood vessel is taken from another part of your body and used to create a new pathway for blood to flow around the blocked artery.

By understanding how your heart works, the causes of heart attacks, and the healing process, you can become more invested in your recovery. Remember, while a scar remains, your heart has the remarkable ability to heal and continue pumping life through your body.

CHAPTER 3: FACING TREATMENT OPTIONS

Partnering with Your Doctor for Recovery

After a heart attack, facing medical interventions can feel overwhelming. This chapter explains different treatment options, helping you understand your role in the recovery process.

Medications for Heart Attack Recovery

Your doctor will likely prescribe medications to address various aspects of your heart health after a heart attack. Here is a breakdown of some common medications:

- **Blood thinners:** These medications help prevent blood clots from forming and blocking arteries. Examples include aspirin and medications like heparin or warfarin.

- **Cholesterol-lowering medications:** Medications like statins help reduce LDL cholesterol levels, slowing down plaque buildup in your arteries.

- **Blood pressure medications:** Medications can help control high blood pressure, reducing the strain on your heart. Examples include diuretics, ACE inhibitors, and beta-blockers.

- **Antianginal medications:** These medications help manage chest pain caused by reduced blood flow to the heart. Nitroglycerin is a common example used during angina attacks.

Understanding the purpose of each medication and taking them as prescribed is crucial for your recovery.

Cardiac Procedures: Unblocking the Arteries

Depending on the severity of the blockage, your doctor might recommend procedures to improve blood flow to the heart muscle. Here are two common approaches:

- **Angioplasty:** During this minimally invasive procedure, a thin catheter (flexible tube) is inserted into a blocked artery. A tiny balloon at the tip of the catheter is inflated to open the blockage. Sometimes, a stent, a small wire mesh tube, is placed in the artery to keep it from narrowing again.

- **Bypass surgery:** In this more complex procedure, a healthy blood vessel from another part of your body is grafted (attached) to create a new pathway for blood to flow around the blocked artery. This improves blood flow to the heart muscle beyond the blockage.

Cardiac Rehabilitation: Getting Back on Track

Cardiac rehabilitation is a crucial part of your recovery journey. It is a personalized program designed to help you regain your strength, improve your heart health, and reduce your risk of future heart problems. These programs typically include:

- **Supervised exercise training:** A healthcare professional will work with you to create a safe and effective exercise plan to improve your heart health and overall fitness.

- **Education:** You will learn about heart disease, risk factors, and how to manage your condition through healthy lifestyle choices.

- **Counseling:** Coping with a heart attack can be emotionally challenging. Cardiac rehabilitation programs often offer support groups or individual counseling to help you manage stress and anxiety.

Remember, you are not alone in navigating these treatment options. Your doctor will work with you to determine the best course of action based on your individual needs.

By actively participating in your treatment plan and following your doctor's recommendations, you can significantly improve your chances of a successful recovery.

PART 2: BUILDING A FOUNDATION FOR A HEALTHY HEART

CHAPTER 4: PARTNERING WITH YOUR DOCTOR

Creating a Personalized Recovery Plan

After a heart attack, recovery is a journey, not a destination. It requires a strong doctor-patient relationship and a personalized plan tailored to your specific needs. This chapter guides you through building a successful partnership with your doctor and creating a recovery plan that empowers you to take control of your health.

Building Trust and Open Communication

A strong doctor-patient relationship is the cornerstone of successful recovery. Here is how to build trust and open communication:

- **Find a doctor you feel comfortable with:** Ask your friends or family for recommendations or research doctors in your area who specialize in heart health. Choose someone you feel comfortable talking to openly and honestly about your concerns.

- **Be an active participant in your care:** Do not hesitate to ask questions and voice your concerns. The more information you share, the better your doctor can understand your situation and create a personalized plan.

- **Come prepared to appointments:** Make a list of questions and track your symptoms, medications, and any concerns you might have.

Understanding Your Risk Factors - A Roadmap for Prevention

Risk factors are like red flags that increase your chances of developing health problems like heart disease. By understanding your individual risk factors, you can work with your doctor to create a personalized plan to address them and prevent future issues.

Here are some common risk factors for heart disease:

- **High blood pressure:** Uncontrolled high blood pressure puts a strain on your heart and arteries.

- **High cholesterol:** Elevated levels of LDL cholesterol contribute to plaque buildup in your arteries.

- **Diabetes:** This chronic condition can damage blood vessels and increase the risk of heart disease.

- **Smoking:** Smoking damages the lining of your arteries and increases your risk of blood clots.

- **Being overweight or obese:** Excess weight puts a strain on your heart and increases your risk of other conditions like diabetes and high blood pressure.

- **Family history:** Having a family history of heart disease increases your risk.

Setting Realistic and Achievable Recovery Goals

Setting realistic and achievable goals is crucial for staying motivated and on track with your recovery. Here is how to approach goal setting:

- **Start small:** Do not try to overhaul your entire lifestyle at once. Begin with small, achievable goals that you can gradually build upon. For example, aiming for a 15-minute walk three times a week might be a good starting point.

- **Focus on progress, not perfection:** Recovery takes time and effort. There might be setbacks along the way. Do not get discouraged; celebrate your progress, no matter how small.

- **Work with your doctor:** Discuss your goals with your doctor. They can help you set realistic and achievable targets based on your individual health and limitations.

Developing a Personalized Recovery Plan

Based on your risk factors, overall health, and recovery goals, your doctor will work with you to create a personalized recovery plan. This plan will likely include:

- **Medications:** Your doctor will prescribe medications to manage your cholesterol, blood pressure, and other heart health concerns.

- **Lifestyle Modifications:** You will likely be advised to make changes to your diet, exercise routine, and stress management habits. This could involve eating a heart-healthy diet, incorporating regular physical activity, and practicing relaxation techniques.

- **Cardiac Rehabilitation:** This comprehensive program can help you strengthen your heart, improve your overall fitness, and learn valuable coping mechanisms.

Remember, you are a partner in your recovery. By building trust with your doctor, understanding your risk factors, and setting realistic goals, you will be empowered to create a personalized recovery plan that gets you back on track to a healthier and happier life.

CHAPTER 5: DIET FOR HEART HEALTH

Nourishing Your Body for Optimal Function

Just like a car needs the right fuel to run smoothly, your heart needs the right nutrients to function optimally. This chapter dives into the principles of a heart-healthy diet, helping you make informed choices that nourish your body and promote recovery after a heart attack.

The Heart-Healthy Diet: A Foundation for Wellbeing

A heart-healthy diet focuses on whole, unprocessed foods that are low in saturated and trans fats, cholesterol, and sodium. It emphasizes foods rich in nutrients that can improve your heart health and overall well-being. Here are some key principles:

- **Focus on Fruits and Vegetables:** Fill your plate with a colorful variety of fruits and vegetables. They're packed with vitamins, minerals, and antioxidants that protect your heart and blood vessels.

- **Choose Whole Grains Over Refined Grains:** Opt for whole grains like brown rice, quinoa, and whole-wheat bread instead of refined grains like white bread and white pasta. Whole grains are higher in fiber, which can help lower cholesterol levels.

- **Select Lean Protein Sources:** Choose lean protein sources like chicken, fish, beans, and lentils over fatty meats. These options provide essential protein without the saturated fat found in red meat.

- **Limit Unhealthy Fats:** Reduce your intake of saturated and trans fats. These fats can increase your LDL cholesterol levels, raising your risk of heart disease.

- **Embrace Healthy Fats:** Include healthy fats from sources like olive oil, avocados, and nuts in your diet. These fats can help lower your LDL cholesterol and raise your HDL cholesterol (the "good" cholesterol).

Making Smart Choices for Your Heart

Here are some practical tips to incorporate these principles into your daily meals:

- **Read Food Labels:** Pay attention to the fat and sodium content when buying packaged foods. Opt for options lower in saturated and trans fats and sodium.

- **Cooking at Home:** Preparing meals at home allows you to control the ingredients and portion sizes. Experiment with heart-healthy recipes that are delicious and satisfying.

- **Limit Added Sugar:** Excessive sugar intake can contribute to weight gain and other health problems. Limit sugary drinks and processed snacks.

- **Do not Forget Hydration:** Staying hydrated is essential for overall health, including heart function. Drink plenty of water throughout the day.

Managing Cholesterol and Blood Pressure Through Diet

Certain dietary choices can significantly impact your cholesterol and blood pressure levels. Here is how food can play a role:

- **Lowering Cholesterol:** Reduce saturated and trans fats and increase fiber intake. Soluble fiber in foods like oats and beans can help trap cholesterol and remove it from your body.

- **Controlling Blood Pressure:** Limit sodium intake. Opt for fresh fruits and vegetables, and choose low-sodium alternatives for packaged foods.

Sample Meal Plans for a Healthy Heart

Creating healthy meal plans does not have to be complicated. Here is a sample daily meal plan to get you started:

- **Breakfast:** Oatmeal with berries and nuts, whole-wheat toast with avocado and eggs.

- **Lunch:** Grilled chicken salad with whole-wheat bread or a veggie wrap with hummus.

- **Dinner:** Salmon with roasted vegetables and brown rice, lentil soup with whole-grain bread.

- **Snacks:** Fruits, nuts, yogurt with granola, vegetable sticks with hummus.

Remember, this is just a sample. You can customize it based on your preferences and dietary needs. There are many resources available with delicious heart-healthy recipes to help you build a menu that's both nutritious and enjoyable.

Following a heart-healthy diet is an investment in your

long-term health. By making informed choices about the food you eat, you can empower your body to recover from a heart attack and live a long, healthy life.

CHAPTER 6: MOVING FORWARD AFTER A HEART ATTACK

Finding Safe and Effective Movement

After a heart attack, the thought of exercise might seem daunting. But regular physical activity is crucial for your recovery and overall well-being. This chapter explains the benefits of exercise after a heart attack and guides you on finding safe and effective ways to get moving again.

The Power of Movement: Why Exercise Matters After a Heart Attack

Regular exercise offers numerous benefits for your heart health after a heart attack:

- **Improves Blood Flow:** Exercise strengthens your heart muscle, allowing it to pump blood more efficiently throughout your body. This improves oxygen delivery to your cells, including those in your heart muscle itself.

- **Lowers Cholesterol:** Physical activity can help lower your LDL cholesterol ("bad" cholesterol) levels and raise your HDL cholesterol ("good" cholesterol) levels, reducing your risk of future heart problems.

- **Controls Blood Pressure:** Exercise can help lower your blood pressure, reducing the strain on your heart and blood vessels.

- **Manages Weight:** Regular physical activity can help you maintain a healthy weight, which further reduces your risk of heart disease.

- **Boosts Mood and Energy Levels:** Exercise releases endorphins, hormones that have mood-boosting and energy-enhancing effects. This can help combat feelings of depression and fatigue after a heart attack.

Finding Your Safe Exercise Zone

Before starting any exercise program, it is crucial to talk to your doctor. They will assess your individual situation and recommend the safest and most effective exercises for you. Here are some general guidelines:

- **Start Slow and Gradually Increase Intensity:** Do not try to overdo it. Begin with low-intensity activities like walking and gradually increase the duration and intensity as your fitness improves.

- **Focus on Cardio and Strength Training:** Aim for at least 150 minutes of moderate-intensity aerobic activity (like brisk walking) or 75 minutes of vigorous-intensity activity (like jogging) per week. Include strength training exercises for major muscle groups at least twice a week.

- **Listen to Your Body:** Pay attention to your body's signals. Stop if you experience chest pain, dizziness, or shortness of breath. These could be signs you are pushing yourself too hard.

Making Movement a Part of Your Day

The key to sticking with an exercise program is finding activities you enjoy. Here are some ideas to incorporate physical activity into your daily routine:

- **Take the Stairs:** Opt for the stairs instead of the elevator whenever possible.

- **Walk During Breaks:** Use your work breaks for short walks instead of sitting at your desk.

- **Park Further Away:** Park further away from your destination and walk the extra distance.

- **Join a Fitness Class:** Consider joining a group exercise class like yoga, water aerobics, or dance fitness.

- **Find an Exercise Buddy:** Having an exercise buddy can help you stay motivated and accountable.

Overcoming Exercise Fears and Limitations

It is natural to have some fear or apprehension about exercise after a heart attack. However, remember that exercise is safe and beneficial when done under proper guidance. Talk to your doctor about your concerns. They can address your fears and work with you to design a program that's safe and effective.

Even with limitations, you can still incorporate physical activity into your life. Here are some tips:

- **Modify Activities:** If certain exercises are difficult, modify them to suit your abilities. For example, you could use a stationary bike instead of going for a run.

- **Focus on Function:** Think about activities that improve your daily life. Simple tasks like gardening or housework can be a form of exercise.

- **Listen to Your Body:** Do not push yourself too hard. Rest when you need to and gradually increase your activity level over time.

Remember, even small amounts of physical activity can

significantly benefit your heart health. By finding safe and enjoyable ways to move your body, you will be well on your way to a stronger, healthier you.

CHAPTER 7: HEALING THROUGH MOVEMENT

Exercise After Heart Surgery

After heart surgery, getting back to your daily activities can feel like a marathon. But incorporating safe and effective exercise into your recovery plan is crucial for strengthening your heart and improving your overall well-being. This chapter explains the importance of exercise after surgery, guides you through safe exercises, and helps you gradually build strength and endurance for a healthier future.

Unique Considerations After Heart Surgery

While similar principles apply to exercise after a heart attack and surgery, there might be additional restrictions based on the type of surgery you underwent. Here are some key things to remember:

- **Post-Surgical Recovery:** Your body needs time to heal after surgery. Your doctor will advise you on specific restrictions and a safe timeline for starting exercise.

- **Understanding Your Limitations:** Be honest with yourself about your physical capabilities after surgery. Do not try to push yourself too hard, and prioritize rest when needed.

Safe Exercises for Post-Surgical Healing

Once your doctor gives you the green light, you can begin incorporating gentle exercises into your routine. Here are some examples of safe activities to promote healing:

- **Walking:** Walking is an excellent low-impact exercise that improves circulation and strengthens your heart muscle. Start with short walks and gradually increase the duration and intensity as tolerated.

- **Stationary Cycling:** This is a great way to exercise your legs without putting too much stress on your joints. You can adjust the resistance to match your fitness level.

- **Swimming:** Water aerobics or gentle swimming offers low-impact exercise while providing cooling benefits.

- **Stretching and Yoga:** Gentle stretching and yoga can improve flexibility and range of motion, aiding in your overall recovery.

Gradually Increasing the Intensity

As your fitness improves, you can gradually increase the intensity of your workouts. However, it is crucial to listen to your body and progress at a safe pace. Here are some tips:

- **Focus on Duration First:** Start by increasing the duration of your workouts before upping the intensity. Aim for longer walks or longer sessions on the stationary bike.

- **Monitor Your Heart Rate:** Talk to your doctor about a safe target heart rate zone for exercise. Use a heart rate monitor to stay within this zone during your workouts.

- **Listen to Your Body:** Pay attention to any pain or discomfort. If you experience any discomfort, slow down or stop the activity and consult your doctor.

Building Long-Term Strength and Endurance:

As you recover and become stronger, you can incorporate more challenging exercises to build long-term strength and endurance. Here is how to gradually build a well-rounded exercise program:

- **Strength Training:** Add strength training exercises using light weights or resistance bands to your routine. This can help improve your overall strength and functional ability.

- **Balance Exercises:** Include simple balance exercises to improve your stability and prevent falls.

- **Cardio Variety:** Once cleared by your doctor, explore other forms of cardio like jogging, dancing, or cycling for a more dynamic workout routine.

Remember, consistency is key. Aim for at least 150 minutes of moderate-intensity aerobic activity or 75 minutes of vigorous-intensity activity per week. Even small increases in activity can significantly benefit your heart health.

Embrace the Journey

Regaining your strength after heart surgery takes time and dedication. Celebrate your progress, no matter how small. Remember, by gradually increasing exercise intensity and incorporating a variety of safe activities, you can build a strong and healthy foundation for long-term well-being.

CHAPTER 8: TAMING THE STRESS TIGER

Techniques for Managing Emotional Wellbeing

A heart attack is not just a physical event; it can take a toll on your emotions. This chapter explores the emotional impact of a heart attack and equips you with tools to manage stress, build resilience, and navigate your emotional journey towards healing.

Facing the Emotional Storm:

After a heart attack, it is normal to experience a wave of emotions like:

- **Anxiety:** You might worry about future health problems or your ability to return to your normal life.

- **Fear:** The experience of the heart attack itself can be frightening, leading to a fear of recurrence.

- **Depression:** Feeling low, down, and losing interest in activities you once enjoyed are common symptoms of depression after a heart attack.

These emotions are valid, and addressing them is crucial for your overall well-being. Here are some techniques to help you manage stress and build resilience:

Relaxation Techniques: Calming the Mind and Body

- **Deep Breathing:** This simple yet powerful technique can significantly reduce stress and anxiety. Focus on slow, deep breaths, inhaling through your nose and exhaling through your mouth.

- **Meditation:** Meditation helps quiet the mind and promote relaxation. There are many guided meditations available online or through apps to help you get started.

- **Progressive Muscle Relaxation:** Tense and relax different muscle groups in your body one by one, focusing on the feeling of relaxation spreading throughout your body.

Building Resilience: A Positive Outlook for Healing

Resilience is your ability to bounce back from challenges. Here is how to cultivate a positive mindset for healing:

- **Focus on Gratitude:** Take time each day to appreciate the good things in your life, even the small things. Gratitude can shift your focus to the positive aspects of your life.

- **Practice Mindfulness:** Mindfulness involves being present in the moment and accepting your thoughts and feelings without judgment. This can help you manage stress and anxiety.

- **Challenge Negative Thoughts:** Our thoughts can influence our emotions. When negative thoughts arise, challenge them with more positive and realistic self-talk.

Seeking Support for Emotional Wellbeing:

You do not have to navigate these emotions alone. Here are some resources that can provide support:

- **Talk Therapy:** Talking to a therapist can provide a safe space to express your emotions and develop coping skills.

- **Support Groups:** Connecting with others who have experienced a heart attack can be incredibly validating and provide a sense of community.

- **Family and Friends:** Talking to your loved ones about your feelings can be a source of comfort and support.

Remember, taking care of your emotional health is just as important as taking care of your physical health. By incorporating relaxation techniques, building resilience, and seeking support, you can manage stress and navigate the emotional road to recovery after a heart attack.

PART 3: RISK FACTOR REDUCTION - A LIFELONG COMMITMENT

CHAPTER 9: CHOLESTEROL CONTROL

Keeping Your Arteries Clear and Healthy

Cholesterol. You might hear this term a lot after a heart attack. This chapter dives into the world of cholesterol, explaining its impact on heart health and how you can manage it through lifestyle changes and medication, if needed.

Understanding the Different Types of Cholesterol

Cholesterol is a waxy substance found in your blood. It is essential for some bodily functions, but high levels can contribute to heart disease. Here is a breakdown of the two main types:

- **LDL Cholesterol (Low-Density Lipoprotein):** Often referred to as "bad" cholesterol. LDL cholesterol builds up in the walls of your arteries, forming plaque. Over time, this plaque can narrow the arteries, reducing blood flow to your heart and increasing your risk of a heart attack.

- **HDL Cholesterol (High-Density Lipoprotein):** Often called "good" cholesterol.

HDL cholesterol helps remove LDL cholesterol from your arteries, preventing plaque buildup.

The Cholesterol Connection to Heart Health

High levels of LDL cholesterol are a significant risk factor for heart disease. When LDL cholesterol accumulates in your arteries, it can form plaque. This plaque narrows the arteries, a condition called atherosclerosis. If a piece of plaque ruptures, it can form a blood clot that completely blocks the artery, leading to a heart attack.

Managing Cholesterol Through Lifestyle Changes

The good news is that you can significantly impact your cholesterol levels through healthy lifestyle choices:

- **Diet:** A heart-healthy diet low in saturated and trans fats, cholesterol, and sodium is crucial. Focus on fruits, vegetables, whole grains, lean protein sources, and healthy fats like those found in olive oil and avocados. (Refer to Chapter 5: Diet for Heart Health for detailed dietary recommendations)

- **Exercise:** Regular physical activity helps lower LDL cholesterol and raise HDL cholesterol. Aim for at least 150 minutes of moderate-intensity exercise or 75 minutes of vigorous-intensity exercise per week. (Refer to Chapter 6: Moving Forward After a Heart Attack and Chapter 7: Heart Surgery for Heart Attack for exercise recommendations after a heart attack or surgery)

- **Weight Management:** Being overweight or obese can contribute to high cholesterol levels. Losing even a moderate amount of weight can significantly improve your cholesterol profile.

- **Smoking Cessation:** Smoking damages your arteries and increases your risk of heart disease. Quitting smoking is one of the best things you can do for your heart health.

Medication Options for Cholesterol Control

If lifestyle changes alone are not enough to manage your cholesterol levels, your doctor might prescribe medication. Here are some common types:

- **Statins:** Statins are the most common type of cholesterol-lowering medication. They work by blocking your liver's production of LDL cholesterol.

- **Ezetimibe:** This medication works by reducing the absorption of cholesterol from your gut.

- **Bile Acid Sequestrants:** These medications bind to cholesterol in your digestive system, allowing it to be eliminated from your body.

Monitoring Your Cholesterol Levels and Staying on Track

Regularly monitoring your cholesterol levels is crucial. Your doctor will recommend how often you should have your blood tested. By keeping track of your cholesterol numbers, you and your doctor can adjust your treatment plan if needed.

Remember, managing cholesterol is a lifelong journey. By combining healthy lifestyle habits with medication, when necessary, you can significantly reduce your risk of future heart problems and keep your arteries clear and healthy.

CHAPTER 10: BLOOD PRESSURE MATTERS

Strategies for Healthy Blood Pressure Levels

Blood pressure. You might get your blood pressure checked at every doctor's visit, but what exactly does it mean? This chapter explains how blood pressure works, its impact on your heart health, and how you can manage it through lifestyle changes and medications, if needed.

Understanding Your Blood Pressure Numbers

Blood pressure is the force exerted by your blood against the walls of your arteries as your heart pumps. It is typically measured in millimeters of mercury (mmHg) with two numbers:

- **Systolic pressure:** This is the top number and represents the pressure when your heart beats.

- **Diastolic pressure:** This is the bottom number and represents the pressure when your heart relaxes between beats.

Healthy versus Unhealthy Blood Pressure Levels

The American Heart Association defines healthy blood pressure as less than 120/80 mmHg. High blood pressure, also known as hypertension, is anything above these levels. Here is a breakdown of blood pressure categories:

- **Normal:** Less than 120/80 mmHg
- **Elevated:** 120-129/80 mmHg (pre-hypertension)
- **Stage 1 Hypertension:** 130-139/80-89 mmHg
- **Stage 2 Hypertension:** 140/90 mmHg or higher

The Silent Threat of High Blood Pressure

High blood pressure often has no symptoms, earning it the nickname "silent killer." Over time, uncontrolled high blood pressure can damage your arteries and increase your risk of:

- Heart attack
- Stroke
- Heart failure
- Kidney disease

Taking Control with Lifestyle Changes

Fortunately, you can significantly impact your blood pressure through healthy lifestyle choices:

- **Diet:** A heart-healthy diet low in sodium, saturated and trans fats, and added sugar is crucial. Focus on fruits, vegetables, whole grains, lean protein sources, and healthy fats. (Refer to Chapter

5: Diet for Heart Health for detailed dietary recommendations).

- **Exercise:** Regular physical activity helps lower blood pressure. Aim for at least 150 minutes of moderate-intensity exercise or 75 minutes of vigorous-intensity exercise per week. (Refer to Chapter 6: Moving Forward After a Heart Attack and Chapter 7: Heart Surgery for Heart Attack for exercise recommendations after a heart attack or surgery).

- **Weight Management:** Losing even a moderate amount of weight can significantly improve your blood pressure.

- **Smoking Cessation:** Smoking damages your arteries and increases your risk of heart disease, including high blood pressure. Quitting smoking is one of the best things you can do for your overall health.

- **Stress Management:** Chronic stress can contribute to high blood pressure. Practice relaxation techniques like deep breathing and meditation to manage stress. (Refer to Chapter 8: Taming the Stress Tiger for relaxation techniques).

- **Limiting Alcohol Consumption:** Excessive alcohol intake can raise your blood pressure.

Medication Options for High Blood Pressure

If lifestyle changes alone are not enough to control your blood pressure, your doctor might prescribe medication. Here are some common types:

- **Diuretics:** These medications help your body get rid of excess fluid through urine, reducing blood volume and lowering pressure.

- **ACE inhibitors:** Angiotensin-converting enzyme (ACE) inhibitors help relax blood vessels, lowering blood pressure.

- **Angiotensin II receptor blockers (ARBs):** These medications work similarly to ACE inhibitors but target a different part of the blood pressure regulation system.

- **Beta-blockers:** Beta-blockers slow down your heart rate and reduce the force of your heart contractions, lowering blood pressure.

Monitoring Your Blood Pressure Regularly

Keeping track of your blood pressure at home is crucial for managing it effectively. Use a home blood pressure monitor and take your readings as directed by your doctor. Regularly monitoring your blood pressure allows you to adjust your lifestyle habits or medications if needed, in consultation with your doctor.

Remember, managing blood pressure is a lifelong commitment. By prioritizing healthy lifestyle habits and taking medication as prescribed, you can significantly reduce your risk of future heart problems and maintain healthy blood pressure levels.

CHAPTER 11: WEIGHT MANAGEMENT

Achieving and Maintaining a Healthy Weight

Weight management plays a crucial role in overall health, especially after a heart attack. This chapter explores the connection between weight and heart health, guides you in setting realistic goals, and provides sustainable strategies to achieve and maintain a healthy weight for a long and healthy life.

Understanding the Weight-Heart Health Connection

Carrying excess weight puts a strain on your heart. Here is how weight can impact your heart health:

- **Increased Blood Pressure:** Excess weight can contribute to high blood pressure, a significant risk factor for heart disease.

- **Elevated Cholesterol Levels:** Being overweight or obese can increase your LDL ("bad") cholesterol and decrease your HDL ("good") cholesterol levels.

- **Risk of Type 2 Diabetes:** Carrying excess weight increases your risk of developing type 2 diabetes, which can further worsen your heart health.

- **Sleep Apnea:** This condition, where breathing repeatedly stops and starts during sleep, is more common in people who are overweight or obese. Sleep apnea can increase your risk of heart attack and stroke.

Setting Realistic and Achievable Goals

Losing weight too quickly is often unsustainable. Here is how to set realistic and achievable goals for weight loss:

- **Focus on Small, Sustainable Changes:** Aim for a gradual weight loss of 1-2 pounds per week. This is a safe and manageable pace for long-term success.

- **Talk to Your Doctor:** Discuss your weight loss goals with your doctor. They can help you set realistic targets based on your individual health and weight.

- **Focus on Progress, Not Perfection:** There might be setbacks along the way. Do not get discouraged; celebrate your progress, no matter how small.

Sustainable Strategies for Weight Management

Reaching and maintaining a healthy weight is a marathon, not a sprint. Here are some sustainable strategies to help you on your journey:

- **Healthy Eating Habits:** Focus on a heart-healthy diet rich in fruits, vegetables, whole grains, and lean protein sources. (Refer to Chapter 5: Diet for Heart Health for detailed dietary recommendations).

- **Portion Control:** Pay attention to portion sizes. Use smaller plates and bowls to avoid overeating.

- **Mindful Eating:** Slow down and savor your food. Eat without distractions and listen to your body's hunger and fullness cues.

- **Increase Physical Activity:** Regular exercise promotes weight loss and helps you maintain a healthy weight. (Refer to Chapter 6: Moving Forward After a Heart Attack and Chapter 7: Heart Surgery for Heart Attack for exercise recommendations after a heart attack or surgery).

- **Stay Hydrated:** Drinking plenty of water throughout the day can help you feel full and reduce cravings.

- **Find a Support System:** Having a friend, family member, or support group can be motivating and keep you accountable on your weight loss journey.

Maintaining a Healthy Weight for Long-Term Health

Losing weight is just the first step. Here is how to maintain a healthy weight for the long term:

- **Make Healthy Habits a Lifestyle:** Do not view your weight loss plan as a temporary fix. Integrate healthy eating and exercise habits into your daily life.

- **Find Activities You Enjoy:** Choose physical activities you enjoy and make them part of your routine. This will make it more likely that you will stick with them.

- **Plan for Setbacks:** Everyone has setbacks. Do not let them derail your progress. Get back on track with your healthy habits and focus on moving forward.

- **Reward Yourself:** Celebrate your achievements on your weight loss journey. This will help you stay motivated and keep you going.

Remember, you are not alone in this journey. With dedication, a healthy weight is achievable. By following these sustainable strategies and maintaining a heart-healthy lifestyle, you can reach and maintain a weight that promotes long-term health and well-being.

CHAPTER 12: SMOKING CESSATION

Breaking Free from the Habit for a Healthier You

Smoking is a major risk factor for heart disease. This chapter dives deep into the dangers of smoking for your heart health, equips you with strategies to develop a quit plan, and highlights the rewards of a smoke-free life.

Smoking: A Threat to Your Heart

Smoking damages your heart and blood vessels in multiple ways:

- **Reduced Blood Flow:** Smoking narrows your arteries by damaging their lining. This reduces blood flow to your heart, increasing your risk of heart attack and stroke.

- **Increased Blood Pressure:** Smoking raises your blood pressure, putting further strain on your heart.

- **Elevated Cholesterol Levels:** Smoking can increase your LDL ("bad") cholesterol and decrease your HDL ("good") cholesterol levels.

- **Blood Clots:** Smoking makes your blood more likely to clot, which can lead to a heart attack or stroke.

Building Your Quit Smoking Plan

Quitting smoking is challenging, but it is one of the best things you can do for your heart health. Here is how to develop a quit plan that works for you:

- **Set a Quit Date:** Choose a specific date in the future when you will stop smoking completely.

- **Identify Your Triggers:** What situations make you crave a cigarette? Stress, social gatherings, or boredom could be triggers. Develop strategies to cope with these triggers without smoking.

- **Consider Nicotine Replacement Therapy:** Nicotine replacement therapy (NRT) products like patches, gum, or lozenges can help manage withdrawal symptoms. Talk to your doctor about the best NRT option for you.

- **Join a Support Group or Quit Smoking Program:** Having a support system can make a big difference. Consider joining a quit smoking program or support group to connect with others who are going through the same journey.

Utilizing Support Systems and Resources

Do not hesitate to utilize available resources to help you quit smoking:

- **Your Doctor:** Talk to your doctor about your quit plan and discuss if medication to help with cravings might be an option.

- **Support Groups:** Online forums, local support groups, or even apps can provide encouragement and connection with others trying to quit.

- **Quitline:** Many regions have free quitlines offering counseling, support, and information.

The Rewards of a Smoke-Free Life

The benefits of quitting smoking are immediate and long-lasting:

- **Improved Heart Health:** Within weeks of quitting, your risk of heart attack starts to decrease.

- **Enhanced Breathing:** You will experience improved lung function and easier breathing.

- **Increased Energy Levels:** Quitting smoking can boost your energy levels and stamina.

- **Reduced Risk of Other Health Problems:** Quitting smoking lowers your risk of cancer, stroke, and other chronic diseases.

- **Improved Sense of Taste and Smell:** Your senses of taste and smell will become sharper after quitting.

Remember, quitting smoking is an investment in your health. Every puff you resist is a step towards a healthier future. By developing a quit plan, utilizing available resources, and focusing on the long-term benefits, you can break free from the grip of smoking and embrace a healthier, smoke-free life.

CHAPTER 13: DIABETES AND HEART HEALTH

Managing Diabetes for a Balanced Heart

Diabetes and heart disease often go hand-in-hand. This chapter explores the connection between these conditions, provides effective diabetes management strategies, and highlights the importance of maintaining healthy blood sugar levels for optimal heart health.

The Diabetes-Heart Disease Connection:

Diabetes, especially type 2 diabetes, significantly increases your risk of heart disease. Here is why:

- **High Blood Sugar:** Chronically high blood sugar levels damage your blood vessels and nerves, increasing your risk of heart attack, stroke, and peripheral artery disease (PAD).

- **Increased Inflammation:** Diabetes can lead to chronic inflammation throughout your body, further contributing to heart disease risk.

- **Unhealthy Cholesterol Levels:** Diabetes can raise your LDL ("bad") cholesterol and lower your HDL ("good") cholesterol levels, creating an unhealthy cholesterol profile.

Effective Diabetes Management Strategies

Managing your diabetes effectively is crucial for protecting your heart health. Here are three key areas to focus on:

- **Diet:** A healthy eating plan that focuses on fruits, vegetables, whole grains, and lean protein sources is essential. Limit processed foods, sugary drinks, and unhealthy fats. (Refer to Chapter 5: Diet for Heart Health for detailed dietary recommendations).

- **Exercise:** Regular physical activity helps lower blood sugar levels and improves overall heart health. Aim for at least 150 minutes of moderate-intensity exercise or 75 minutes of vigorous-intensity exercise per week. (Refer to Chapter 6: Moving Forward After a Heart Attack and Chapter 7: Heart Surgery for Heart Attack for exercise recommendations after a heart attack or surgery). If you have diabetes, discuss a safe exercise plan with your doctor.

- **Medication:** If lifestyle changes alone are not enough to control your blood sugar levels, your doctor might prescribe medication. These medications can help your body produce or use insulin more effectively.

Maintaining Healthy Blood Sugar Levels

Keeping your blood sugar levels within the target range set by your doctor is crucial for protecting your heart. Here are some tips:

- **Monitor Your Blood Sugar Regularly:** Regularly check your blood sugar levels as directed by your doctor. This helps you understand how your body reacts to food, exercise, and medication.

- **Learn About Carb Counting:** Carbohydrates significantly impact blood sugar levels. Understanding carb counting can help you make informed food choices and manage your blood sugar.

- **Take Medication as Prescribed:** If you are on medication, take it exactly as prescribed by your doctor. Skipping doses can lead to uncontrolled blood sugar levels.

Working with Your Doctor for Optimal Diabetes Control

Your doctor is your partner in managing your diabetes. Here is how to work effectively with them for optimal diabetes control:

- **Regular Checkups:** Attend all your scheduled appointments with your doctor. This allows them to monitor your blood sugar levels, adjust your treatment plan as needed, and address any concerns you might have.

- **Open Communication:** Be open and honest with your doctor about your blood sugar levels, any challenges you face with managing your diabetes, and any questions you may have.

- **Collaboration is Key:** Work together with your doctor to create a personalized diabetes management plan that fits your lifestyle and needs.

Remember, managing diabetes is a lifelong journey. By prioritizing healthy habits, taking your medication as prescribed, and working closely with your doctor, you can effectively manage your diabetes and protect your heart health.

PART 4: LIVING A FULFILLING LIFE AFTER A HEART ATTACK

CHAPTER 14: RETURNING TO WORK AND ACTIVITY

Balancing Work, Rest, and Recovery

Returning to work after a heart attack can be both exciting and daunting. This chapter guides you through a smooth transition back to your professional life, emphasizing the importance of balancing work demands with rest and recovery for optimal healing.

A Gradual Return to Routine

The timeline for returning to work after a heart attack varies depending on the severity of your condition and your job demands. Your doctor will advise you on a safe and gradual return-to-work plan. This might involve starting with part-time hours and gradually increasing your workload as your strength and stamina improve.

Setting Boundaries and Managing Work Stress

Work can be a significant source of stress. Here is how to set boundaries and manage stress at work:

- **Communicate with Your Employer:** Talk to your employer about your limitations and the need for a modified work schedule or adjustments to your workload. Most employers are understanding and can accommodate your needs during recovery.

- **Learn to Say No:** Do not be afraid to politely decline additional tasks or responsibilities if you feel overwhelmed. Focus on completing your current tasks effectively, prioritizing your health and recovery.

- **Take Breaks Regularly:** Get up and move around throughout the day. Take short walks or stretching breaks to prevent fatigue and maintain focus.

- **Practice Relaxation Techniques:** Deep breathing exercises or mindfulness meditation can help you manage stress in the workplace. (Refer to Chapter 8: Taming the Stress Tiger for relaxation techniques).

Balancing Work with Rest and Recovery

While returning to work is important, prioritizing rest and recovery is crucial for healing. Here is how to strike a balance:

- **Listen to Your Body:** Pay attention to your energy levels. Take breaks when you feel tired, and do not push yourself too hard.

- **Schedule Time for Relaxation:** Make time for activities you enjoy outside of work. Relaxation helps reduce stress and promotes healing.

- **Maintain a Healthy Sleep Schedule:** Aim for 7-8 hours of quality sleep each night. Adequate sleep is essential for both physical and mental recovery.

- **Maintain a Healthy Diet:** Continue prioritizing a heart-healthy diet rich in fruits, vegetables, and whole grains. (Refer to Chapter 5: Diet for Heart Health for detailed dietary recommendations).

The Power of Open Communication

Open communication with your employer is vital for a smooth transition back to work. Here is why:

- **Understanding Your Needs:** Discussing your limitations and recovery process with your employer allows them to support you better.

- **Creating a Supportive Environment:** An understanding and supportive work environment can significantly contribute to your well-being during recovery.

- **Building Trust:** Open communication fosters trust between you and your employer, creating a positive work experience.

Remember, returning to work after a heart attack is a journey, not a destination. By prioritizing rest and recovery, setting boundaries at work, and communicating openly with your employer, you can achieve a healthy balance and successfully reintegrate into your professional life.

CHAPTER 15: SLEEP AND HEART HEALTH

The Importance of Quality Sleep

Ever heard the saying "sleep on it"? Well, when it comes to your heart health, a good night's sleep is more than just a saying; it is essential. This chapter explores the link between sleep and heart health, provides strategies for improving sleep quality, and helps you establish a healthy sleep routine for optimal well-being.

Why Sleep Matters for Your Heart

Just like any other muscle in your body, your heart needs time to rest and repair itself. Here is how sleep impacts your heart health:

- **Cellular Repair:** During sleep, your body repairs tissues, and cells throughout your body, including those in your heart.

- **Blood Pressure Regulation:** When you sleep, your blood pressure naturally dips. Chronic sleep deprivation can lead to consistently high blood pressure, a risk factor for heart disease.

- **Inflammation Control:** Sleep helps regulate your body's inflammatory response. Chronic sleep problems can contribute to inflammation, which is linked to an increased risk of heart disease.

Strategies for a Better Night's Sleep

Creating a healthy sleep environment and practicing good sleep hygiene can significantly improve your sleep quality. Here are some tips:

- **Create a Relaxing Bedtime Routine:** Wind down before bed with calming activities like taking a warm bath, reading a book, or practicing relaxation techniques. (Refer to Chapter 8: Taming the Stress Tiger for relaxation techniques).

- **Establish a Regular Sleep Schedule:** Go to bed and wake up at consistent times each day, even on weekends. This helps regulate your body's natural sleep-wake cycle.

- **Optimize Your Sleep Environment:** Ensure your bedroom is dark, quiet, cool, and clutter-free. Invest in a comfortable mattress and pillows.

- **Limit Screen Time Before Bed:** The blue light emitted from electronic devices can disrupt your sleep cycle. Avoid screens for at least an hour before bedtime.

- **Regular Exercise:** Regular physical activity can improve sleep quality. However, avoid strenuous exercise close to bedtime as it can be stimulating.

- **Relaxing Bath:** A warm bath before bed can help you relax and unwind, promoting better sleep.

Overcoming Sleep Problems After a Heart Attack

Sometimes, after a heart attack, you might experience sleep problems due to anxiety, medication side effects, or pain. Here are some tips to manage these challenges:

- **Talk to Your Doctor:** Discuss your sleep problems with your doctor. They might be able to adjust your medication or recommend treatments to address any underlying issues.

- **Cognitive Behavioral Therapy (CBT):** CBT can help identify and change negative thoughts and behaviors that might be interfering with your sleep.

Establishing a Healthy Sleep Routine

Getting on a consistent sleep schedule is crucial for good sleep hygiene. Here is how to create a healthy sleep routine:

- **Set a Regular Bedtime and Wake-Up Time:** Choose a bedtime and wake-up time that allows you to get 7-8 hours of sleep each night. Stick to this schedule as much as possible, even on weekends.

- **Create a Relaxing Bedtime Routine:** Develop a calming routine before bed that signals to your body it is time to wind down. This could include taking a warm bath, reading a book, or practicing relaxation techniques.

- **Avoid Stimulants Before Bed:** Limit caffeine and alcohol intake, especially in the hours leading up to bedtime. Both can disrupt your sleep.

- **Make Sure Your Bedroom is Sleep-Friendly:** Ensure your bedroom is dark, quiet, cool, and clutter-free. This creates a comfortable environment that promotes sleep.

- **See Sunlight During the Day:** Getting some natural sunlight exposure during the day can help regulate your body's natural sleep-wake cycle.

Remember, prioritizing sleep is an investment in your overall health.

By establishing a healthy sleep routine and addressing

any underlying sleep problems, you can improve your sleep quality and support optimal heart health.

CHAPTER 16: BUILDING RESILIENCE

Managing the Emotional Aftermath of a Heart Attack

A heart attack is not just a physical event; it can take a toll on your emotions. This chapter explores the emotional rollercoaster you might be on after a heart attack and equips you with tools to build resilience and navigate your path towards healing.

Facing the Emotional Storm

It is normal to experience a wave of emotions after a heart attack. You might be feeling:

- **Fear:** The experience of the heart attack itself can be frightening, leading to a fear of recurrence.

- **Anxiety:** You might worry about future health problems or your ability to return to your normal life.

- **Depression:** Feeling low, down, and losing interest in activities you once enjoyed are common symptoms of depression after a heart attack.

These emotions are valid, and addressing them is crucial for your overall well-being. Here are some healthy ways to manage these emotions:

- **Talk to Someone You Trust:** Sharing your feelings with a friend, family member, therapist, or support group can be incredibly validating and provide emotional support.

- **Express Yourself Creatively:** Journaling, painting, or playing music can be healthy outlets for expressing your emotions.

- **Practice Relaxation Techniques:** Deep breathing, mindfulness meditation, or progressive muscle relaxation can help calm your mind and body, reducing anxiety and promoting emotional well-being. (Refer to Chapter 8: Taming the Stress Tiger for relaxation techniques).

Building a Strong Support System

You do not have to navigate these emotions alone. Here are some resources that can provide support:

- **Family and Friends:** Talking to your loved ones about your feelings can be a source of comfort and understanding.

- **Support Groups:** Connecting with others who have experienced a heart attack can be incredibly validating and provide a sense of community.

- **Therapy:** Talking to a therapist can provide a safe space to express your emotions and develop coping skills.

Finding Strength in Support and Therapy

Support groups and therapy can be particularly beneficial for managing the emotional aftermath of a heart attack:

- **Support Groups:** Connecting with others who understand what you are going through can reduce feelings of isolation and provide valuable advice and encouragement.

- **Therapy:** A therapist can help you identify negative thought patterns, develop coping mechanisms for stress and anxiety, and promote emotional healing.

The Power of Positive Thinking and Self-Compassion

Developing a positive outlook and practicing self-compassion are essential for building resilience:

- **Positive Thinking:** Focusing on gratitude for the good things in your life and setting realistic goals for recovery can improve your mood and outlook.

- **Self-Compassion:** Be kind to yourself. Acknowledge the challenges you are facing and focus on progress, not perfection.

Remember, building resilience is a journey. By acknowledging and expressing your emotions, leaning on your support system, and incorporating healthy coping mechanisms, you can navigate the emotional challenges after a heart attack and emerge stronger and more resilient.

CHAPTER 17: THE POWER OF SUPPORT

Building a Strong Support Network

After a heart attack, the road to recovery goes beyond medication and lifestyle changes. Social connection and a strong support network are crucial for your emotional and mental well-being. This chapter dives into the importance of support, how to identify and build upon it, and its role in your overall recovery journey.

The Strength of Social Connection

Humans are social creatures, and social connection is essential for overall health. Here is how a strong support network can benefit you after a heart attack:

- **Emotional Support:** Talking to loved ones or support groups provides a safe space to express your emotions, anxieties, and fears. This emotional validation can significantly reduce stress and promote healing.

- **Motivation and Encouragement:** A supportive network can be your cheerleader, motivating you to stick to your healthy lifestyle changes and recovery plan.

- **Reduced Loneliness and Isolation:** Feeling isolated can worsen your emotional state. A strong support network combats loneliness and fosters a sense of belonging.

- **Improved Quality of Life:** Social connections bring joy and laughter into your life, contributing to a better overall well-being.

Identifying Your Support System

Look around you – your support system is likely already there:

- **Family and Friends:** Close friends and family members who care about you and are willing to listen are invaluable sources of support.

- **Partners and Spouses:** Your partner can be a pillar of strength, offering emotional support and practical help during your recovery.

- **Neighbors and Community Members:** Do not underestimate the power of good neighbors or community members who can offer companionship and assistance when needed.

Building Bridges of Communication

Sometimes, letting people support you requires clear

communication. Here is how to ask for help:

- **Be Open About Your Needs:** Do not be afraid to express what you need, whether it is emotional support, help with daily tasks, or just someone to listen.

- **Specific Requests:** Instead of saying "I need help," be specific. "Could you accompany me to my doctor's appointment?" or "Would you mind picking up some groceries?" are clear requests that people can easily fulfill.

- **Practice Gratitude:** Thank your support system for their time, effort, and care. Showing appreciation strengthens the bond and encourages continued support.

Expanding Your Support Network

There are additional avenues to expand your support network beyond your immediate circle:

- **Healthcare Professionals:** Your doctor, nurses, and cardiac rehabilitation team are there to support your recovery. Do not hesitate to ask them questions or express any concerns you might have.

- **Support Groups:** Connecting with others who have experienced a heart attack can be incredibly beneficial. Support groups provide a safe space to share experiences, learn from others, and feel less alone. There are online and in-person support groups available depending on your preference.

- **Therapy:** A therapist can provide individual support, helping you navigate the emotional challenges after a heart attack and develop coping mechanisms.

Remember, building a strong support network is an ongoing process. By identifying your existing support system, communicating your needs clearly, and exploring additional avenues for connection, you can create a powerful network that fosters your emotional well-being and empowers you on your road to recovery.

CHAPTER 18: SEX AND INTIMACY AFTER A HEART ATTACK

Rekindling Intimacy

A heart attack can affect your life in many ways, and intimacy with your partner might be a concern. This chapter explores the physical and emotional impact of a heart attack on intimacy, emphasizes the importance of open communication, and guides you on a gradual return to sexual activity.

The Heart-Intimacy Connection

A heart attack can impact intimacy in two ways:

- **Physical Changes:** After a heart attack, you might experience fatigue, shortness of breath, or limitations due to medication. These physical changes can affect your energy levels and desire for intimacy.

- **Emotional Impact:** The emotional rollercoaster after a heart attack can lead to anxiety, depression, or fear of recurrence. These emotions can affect your mood and libido, impacting intimacy.

Open Communication is Key

Talking openly and honestly with your partner is

crucial for navigating intimacy after a heart attack. Here is how communication can help:

- **Understanding Each Other's Needs:** Share your concerns and limitations openly with your partner. Listen to their concerns as well. This fosters empathy and helps you find ways to reconnect emotionally and physically.

- **Managing Expectations:** Be realistic about your recovery timeline. Discuss a gradual return to intimacy that is comfortable for both of you.

- **Finding Alternatives:** Explore non-sexual ways to express intimacy, such as cuddling, holding hands, or spending quality time together.

A Gradual Return to Intimacy

Focus on rediscovering intimacy at your own pace. Here are some tips for a gradual return to sexual activity:

- **Get Your Doctor's Approval:** Talk to your doctor about when it is safe to resume sexual activity. They can address any concerns you might have and provide guidance based on your individual situation.

- **Start Slowly:** Do not rush back into vigorous sexual activity. Begin with gentle touching and gradually increase intimacy as you feel comfortable.

- **Listen to Your Body:** Pay attention to your body's signals. If you experience any pain, shortness of breath, or discomfort, stop the activity and talk to your doctor.

Seeking Professional Help (if needed)

Sometimes, physical or emotional challenges can persist and affect your sexual life. Do not hesitate to seek professional help:

- **Sex Therapy:** A sex therapist can help address any sexual concerns you or your partner might have and develop strategies for a fulfilling sexual life after a heart attack.

- **Cardiologist or Primary Care Physician:** Your doctor can address any physical concerns that might be impacting your sexual function.

Remember, intimacy is about more than just sex. It is about connection, communication, and feeling loved and supported. By prioritizing open communication, focusing on a gradual return to intimacy, and seeking professional help if needed, you can rebuild intimacy with your partner and experience a fulfilling relationship after a heart attack.

PART 5: LOOKING FORWARD - A LIFETIME OF HEART HEALTH

CHAPTER 19: PREVENTION IS KEY

Strategies for Long-Term Heart Health

Congratulations on taking charge of your heart health. This chapter focuses on how to make those positive changes you have implemented a way of life, ensuring a healthy heart for years to come.

Keeping Your Heart Healthy:

By prioritizing healthy habits, you can significantly reduce your risk of heart disease and live a long and fulfilling life. Here are some key strategies for long-term heart health:

- **Maintain a Healthy Diet:** Continue prioritizing a heart-healthy diet rich in fruits, vegetables, whole grains, and lean protein sources. Limit processed foods, sugary drinks, and unhealthy fats.

- **Regular Exercise:** Aim for at least 150 minutes of moderate-intensity exercise or 75 minutes of vigorous-intensity exercise per week. Find activities you enjoy and make them part of your routine.

- **Maintain a Healthy Weight:** Being overweight or obese increases your risk of heart disease. If you need to lose weight, focus on gradual, sustainable weight loss.

- **Manage Stress:** Chronic stress can raise your blood pressure and contribute to heart disease. Practice relaxation techniques like deep breathing, meditation, or yoga to manage stress. (Refer to Chapter 8: Taming the Stress Tiger for relaxation techniques).

- **Do not Smoke:** Smoking is a major risk factor for heart disease. If you smoke, quitting is the single best thing you can do for your heart health. (Refer to Chapter 12: Smoking Cessation for strategies to quit smoking).

- **Limit Alcohol Consumption:** Excessive alcohol consumption can increase your blood pressure and risk of heart disease.

- **Get Enough Sleep:** Aim for 7-8 hours of quality sleep each night. Adequate sleep plays a crucial role in overall health, including heart health. (Refer to Chapter 15: Sleep and Heart Health for tips on improving sleep quality).

Regular Checkups and Preventive Screenings

Regular checkups with your doctor are vital for monitoring your heart health and identifying any potential problems early on. These checkups might include:

- **Blood Pressure Monitoring:** High blood pressure is a major risk factor for heart disease. Regular monitoring allows your doctor to adjust medication if needed and ensure your blood pressure is under control.

- **Cholesterol Checks:** High blood cholesterol levels can increase your risk of heart attack and stroke. Regular cholesterol checks allow your doctor to monitor your levels and recommend dietary or medication changes if needed.

- **Blood Sugar Monitoring:** Diabetes is a significant risk factor for heart disease. If you have diabetes, regular blood sugar monitoring is essential for managing your condition.

Identifying and Addressing New Risk Factors:

As you age or your lifestyle changes, new risk factors for heart disease might emerge. Here is how to stay vigilant:

- **Be Aware of Family History:** Talk to your doctor about your family history of heart disease. Knowing your risk factors can help your doctor create a personalized preventive plan.

- **Open Communication with Your Doctor:** Discuss any new symptoms or changes in your health with your doctor. This allows them to identify and address any potential problems early on.

- **Regular Screenings:** Follow your doctor's recommendations for preventive screenings, such as EKGs (electrocardiograms) or stress tests, to monitor your heart health.

Living a Heart-Healthy Lifestyle

Making heart-healthy choices a way of life is crucial for long-term well-being. Here are some additional tips:

- **Find Activities You Enjoy:** Choose physical activities you find enjoyable so they become a sustainable part of your routine.

- **Cook More at Home:** Cooking at home allows you to control the ingredients in your meals, making healthier choices easier.

- **Read Food Labels:** Pay attention to nutrition labels when you buy packaged foods. Choose options low in saturated and trans fats, sodium, and added sugars.

- **Manage Stress Effectively:** Chronic stress can negatively impact your heart health. Develop healthy coping mechanisms to manage stress effectively.

Travel Tips for a Healthy Heart

Traveling should not disrupt your healthy habits. Here are some tips for maintaining a heart-healthy lifestyle on the go:

- **Pack Healthy Snacks:** Pack healthy snacks like fruits, nuts, or whole-grain crackers to avoid unhealthy options during travel.

- **Stay Hydrated:** Drink plenty of water throughout your travels to stay hydrated and prevent fatigue.

- **Maintain Activity Levels:** Find ways to stay active while traveling, such as taking walking tours, exploring new places on foot, or using hotel gyms.

- **Be Mindful of Food Choices:** Traveling often involves eating out more. Choose restaurants that offer healthy options or opt for smaller portions.

Remember, prevention is key to a healthy heart. By prioritizing healthy habits, attending regular checkups, and remaining vigilant about your health, you can significantly reduce your risk of heart disease

CHAPTER 20: STAYING MOTIVATED

Maintaining a Healthy Lifestyle Over Time

Making healthy changes is fantastic. But staying motivated and making those changes a permanent part of your life can be challenging. This chapter equips you with strategies to maintain a healthy lifestyle over time, keeping you on the path to long-term well-being.

Setting SMART Goals

Goals are crucial for motivation, but unrealistic goals can lead to frustration and discouragement. Here is how to set SMART goals for lasting success:

- **Specific:** Instead of saying "I want to be healthier," define what "healthier" means for you. Aim for "I will walk for 30 minutes three times a week."

- **Measurable:** Track your progress. Use a pedometer for your walks or a food journal to monitor your diet.

- **Attainable:** Do not try to change everything at once. Start with small, achievable goals that you can gradually build upon.

- **Relevant:** Make sure your goals align with your overall health goals and lifestyle.

- **Time-bound:** Set a timeframe for reaching your goals. This creates a sense of urgency and accomplishment.

Finding Activities You Love

Exercise and healthy eating should not feel like punishment. Here is how to make healthy choices enjoyable:

- **Discover Your Passions:** Do you like dancing? Swimming? Find physical activities you genuinely enjoy. You are more likely to stick with them if you have fun.

- **Explore Different Cuisines:** Healthy eating does not have to be bland. Experiment with recipes from different cultures to discover delicious and nutritious meals.

- **Turn it into a Social Activity:** Cooking with friends or family, joining a walking group, or taking a fitness class together can add a social element to your healthy habits.

Building a Support System for Motivation

A strong support system can be your biggest cheerleader. Here is how to leverage your support network:

- **Share Your Goals:** Tell your family, friends, or a support group about your health goals. Their encouragement can make a big difference.

- **Find an Accountability Partner:** Partner up with a friend who also wants to live a healthier lifestyle. Hold each other accountable and celebrate successes together.

- **Join Online Communities:** There are online communities and forums dedicated to healthy living. Connect with others for inspiration, tips, and support.

Rewarding Yourself

Celebrating your achievements is a great way to stay motivated. Here is how to reward yourself:

- **Non-Food Rewards:** Plan rewards that do not revolve around food. Treat yourself to a massage, a new book, or an activity you enjoy.

- **Milestone Rewards:** Celebrate reaching specific milestones in your journey. This reinforces positive behavior and keeps you motivated.

- **Focus on Progress:** Do not wait for perfection to celebrate. Acknowledge your progress, no matter how small, to keep yourself motivated.

Remember, maintaining a healthy lifestyle is a journey, not a destination. There will be setbacks and challenges. But by setting realistic goals, finding joy in healthy habits, leveraging your support system, and rewarding yourself, you can stay motivated and make healthy choices a permanent part of your life.

CHAPTER 21: CELEBRATING SUCCESS

Recognizing and Appreciating Your Achievements

Taking charge of your heart health is an incredible feat. This chapter delves into the importance of self-acknowledgment and celebration. We will explore ways to track your progress, appreciate your commitment, and cultivate a positive outlook for continued success.

The Power of Self-Appreciation

Taking care of your heart requires dedication and effort. Here is why acknowledging your achievements is essential:

- **Boosts Motivation:** Celebrating your victories, big or small, fuels motivation to keep moving forward on your health journey.

- **Improves Self-Esteem:** Recognizing your accomplishments fosters a sense of pride and confidence in your ability to make and maintain healthy changes.

- **Reduces Stress:** Taking the time to appreciate your efforts can help alleviate stress and promote overall well-being.

Tracking Your Progress - Milestones Mark the Way

Monitoring your progress provides tangible evidence of your hard work. Here is how tracking your progress can be motivating:

- **Journaling:** Keeping a journal allows you to track your accomplishments, challenges, and overall progress over time.

- **Fitness Trackers:** Wearable devices can track your activity levels, sleep patterns, and other health metrics, providing valuable data on your progress.

- **Health Apps:** Utilize apps to monitor your diet, exercise routines, and weight management.

Taking Pride in Your Commitment

Living a heart-healthy life requires commitment, even on days when motivation might dip. Here is why taking pride in your commitment is important:

- **Acknowledge Every Step:** Celebrate not just major milestones but also the everyday choices you make towards a healthier life.

- **Focus on the Journey:** While reaching goals is rewarding, appreciate the effort you put in every day to make healthy choices.

- **You Are Enough:** There will be slip-ups. Do not beat yourself up. Celebrate your commitment to getting back on track.

Maintaining a Positive and Grateful Outlook

A positive outlook empowers you to handle challenges and keep moving forward. Here is how to cultivate gratitude and positivity:

- **Focus on the Benefits:** Shift your mindset. Instead of seeing healthy habits as restrictions, focus on how they make you feel better and improve your overall health.

- **Practice Gratitude:** Take some time each day to appreciate the positive changes you have made and the benefits you are experiencing.

- **Visualize Success:** Imagine yourself reaching your goals and living a healthy life. Visualization can be a powerful tool for motivation.

Remember, celebrating success is not an indulgence; it

is a necessity. Taking the time to acknowledge your achievements, big and small, fuels your motivation, reinforces positive habits, and empowers you to continue your journey towards a healthy heart. Congratulations on taking charge of your well-being.

CHAPTER 22: LIVING WITH GRATITUDE

Embracing a Life Well Lived

A heart attack can be a life-altering event. But within that challenge lies an opportunity. This chapter explores the power of gratitude for improved well-being and guides you on cultivating a grateful heart, finding joy and purpose, and embracing a fulfilling life after a heart attack.

The Magic of Gratitude

Gratitude is not just a nice feeling; it is a powerful tool for improving your overall well-being. Here is how:

- **Boosts Happiness:** Appreciating the good things in your life elevates your mood and promotes feelings of happiness and contentment.

- **Reduces Stress:** Focusing on gratitude can shift your perspective away from stress and negativity, fostering a sense of calm and well-being.

- **Strengthens Relationships:** Expressing gratitude to those who support you strengthens your connections and fosters deeper bonds.

Weaving Gratitude into Your Day

Gratitude does not require grand gestures. Here are simple ways to incorporate gratitude into your daily life:

- **Start a Gratitude Journal:** Dedicate a few minutes each day to write down things you are grateful for, big or small.

- **Practice Mindfulness:** Take a moment to appreciate the simple things around you – a beautiful sunset, a warm cup of coffee, the laughter of a loved one.

- **Express Appreciation:** Tell your loved ones how much you appreciate their presence and support.

Finding Joy and Purpose After a Heart Attack:

A heart attack might make you re-evaluate your life. Here is how to rediscover joy and purpose:

- **Explore New Interests:** Have you always wanted to try painting, dancing, or learning a new language? Now is the perfect time to explore new passions and add joy to your life.

- **Volunteer Your Time:** Giving back to the community can be incredibly fulfilling. Find a cause you care about and volunteer your time and talents.

- **Spend Time with Loved Ones:** Nurture your relationships with family and friends. Spending quality time with loved ones brings joy and strengthens your support system.

Living a Fulfilling and Heart-Healthy Life

Taking care of your heart allows you to live a long and fulfilling life. Here is how to combine a heart-healthy lifestyle with a joyful and meaningful existence:

- **Focus on Experiences, Not Possessions:** Prioritize experiences and creating memories with loved ones over material things.

- **Live in the Moment:** Savor the present moment instead of dwelling on the past or worrying about the future.

- **Set New Goals:** Having goals to work towards provides a sense of purpose and keeps you motivated.

Remember, gratitude is a journey, not a destination. By incorporating gratitude practices into your life, finding joy in everyday moments, and living with purpose, you can experience a deeper sense of well-being and embrace a life well lived after a heart attack. You are a survivor, and your future is full of possibilities.

CHAPTER 23: EMPOWERING YOURSELF WITH KNOWLEDGE

Additional Resources for Continued Learning

Congratulations on taking charge of your heart health. Knowledge is power, and this chapter equips you with valuable resources to continue learning and staying informed about your heart health.

Exploring the Digital Landscape

The internet offers a wealth of information on heart health. Here is how to find reliable online resources:

- **Government Websites:** Government health agencies like the National Institutes of Health (NIH) or the Centers for Disease Control and Prevention (CDC) offer trustworthy and up-to-date information on heart disease, prevention, and treatment.

- **Heart Health Organizations:** Reputable organizations like the American Heart Association (AHA) or the American College of Cardiology (ACC) provide a wealth of resources, including articles, videos, and educational materials on various heart health topics.

- **Online Support Groups:** Connecting with online communities of heart disease survivors or people managing heart conditions can be a source of information, encouragement, and shared experiences. Remember to be critical of information found online and consult your doctor with any questions you may have.

Beyond the Screen: Books and Educational Materials:

- **Heart Health Books:** Numerous books written by medical professionals or heart disease survivors offer in-depth information and practical advice on managing heart health. Ask your doctor for recommendations or visit your local library.

- **Educational Brochures and Pamphlets:** Many hospitals, clinics, and heart health organizations offer free brochures and pamphlets on various heart conditions and healthy lifestyle practices.

Building a Support Network

- **Support Groups:** Joining a local heart disease support group can be an invaluable resource. Sharing experiences, learning from others, and receiving encouragement can be incredibly beneficial.

- **Community Programs:** Many communities offer heart health awareness programs, cooking classes focused on heart-healthy meals, or exercise programs designed for individuals with heart conditions.

Your Doctor - A Partner in Your Health

- **Regular Checkups:** Routine checkups and appointments with your doctor are crucial for monitoring your heart health, addressing any concerns promptly, and staying informed about the latest advancements in preventive care and treatment options.

- **Ask Questions:** Do not hesitate to ask your doctor questions about your heart health, medications, or lifestyle changes. The more informed you are, the better equipped you are to manage your health.

Remember, lifelong learning is key to maintaining good heart health. By utilizing the resources provided in this chapter and actively engaging with your doctor, you can empower yourself with knowledge, stay informed, and make informed decisions about your health and well-being.

Resources

Here is a list of reliable resources on heart attack information from various countries, ensuring a global perspective on this critical health issue:

United States

- American Heart Association (AHA)
  Website: [heart.org]
  Description: Provides comprehensive information on heart attacks, including symptoms, prevention, and treatment options.

- Centers for Disease Control and Prevention (CDC)
  Website:[cdc.gov/heartdisease]
  Description: Offers detailed data and resources on heart disease and heart attacks, including statistics, risk factors, and prevention strategies.

United Kingdom

- British Heart Foundation (BHF)
  Website: [bhf.org.uk]
  Description: A leading charity providing extensive information on heart attacks, research, patient support, and healthy living tips.

- NHS (National Health Service)
  Website: [nhs.uk/conditions/heart-attack]
  Description: The UK's publicly funded healthcare system offering detailed information on heart attack symptoms, treatment, and recovery.

Canada

- Heart and Stroke Foundation of Canada
  Website: [heartandstroke.ca]
  Description: Provides resources on heart disease and stroke, including heart attack symptoms, emergency response, and prevention tips.

- Canadian Cardiovascular Society (CCS)
  Website: [ccs.ca]
  Description: A professional association offering guidelines, research, and information on cardiovascular health, including heart attacks.

Australia

- Heart Foundation of Australia
  Website: [heartfoundation.org.au]
  Description: Offers extensive information on heart disease, including heart attacks, prevention, treatment, and research initiatives.

India

- Indian Heart Association (IHA)
  Website: [indianheartassociation.org]
  Description: Focuses on raising awareness and providing information about heart disease and heart attacks in India.

European Union

- European Society of Cardiology (ESC)
  Website: [escardio.org]
  Description: Provides a wide range of information on cardiovascular diseases, including heart attacks, research, guidelines, and educational resources.

Japan

- Japanese Circulation Society (JCS)
  Website: [j-circ.or.jp]
  Description: Offers information on cardiovascular diseases, including heart attacks, with a focus on research and clinical practice guidelines in Japan.

Global

- World Heart Federation (WHF)
  Website: [world-heart-federation.org]
  Description: An international organization providing global leadership in cardiovascular

health, including resources and advocacy on heart attacks.

These resources provide comprehensive, up-to-date information on heart attacks, from symptoms and risk factors to treatment and prevention strategies, catering to both the general public and healthcare professionals.

Can You Help Others Find This Book by Writing a Review?

Thank you for reading the book. As a retired physician with a fresh viewpoint, I am dedicating my time to creating this informative series out of a desire to empower others through credible information. This series is my way of continuing to serve others, not for profit, but out of a deep love and passion for sharing knowledge to benefit those who are perplexed by the overwhelming information overload in the digital world. Therefore, I have created this series of patient information books as a one-stop information haven, painstakingly built to save you valuable time. Your honest review on Amazon, accessible through the QR code below, will be a guiding light for others seeking clarity. Let us empower each other, one informed reader at a time! Kindly write a review about this book!

ABOUT THE AUTHOR

Dr. A. Mitra is a retired medical doctor who has worked in the field of General Practice in Family Medicine in India and Australia for over 30 years. He completed his graduate education in India and then did further studies in Australia and UK. Currently he lives a private modest life and pursues his interests in reading and writing on various topics.

Printed in Dunstable, United Kingdom